Water Purification For Survival

A Guide for Purification and Conservation of Water

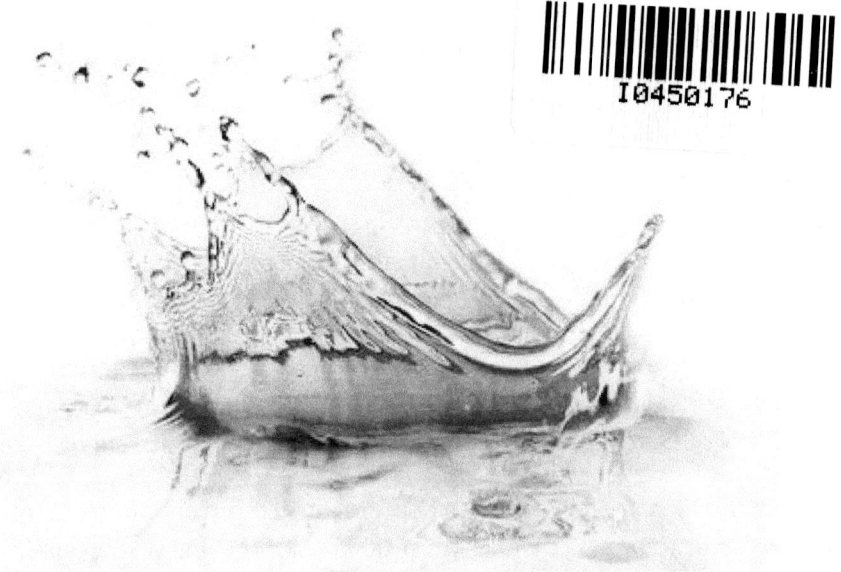

Prepping and Survival Series

M. Usman

Mendon Cottage Books

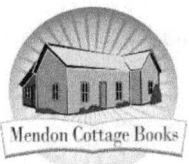

JD-Biz Publishing

Disclaimer

The information is this book is provided for informational purposes only. It is not intended to be used and medical advice or a substitute for proper medical treatment by a qualified health care provider. The information is believed to be accurate as presented based on research by the author.

The contents have not been evaluated by the U.S. Food and Drug Administration or any other Government or Health Organization and the contents in this book are not to be used to treat cure or prevent disease.

The author or publisher is not responsible for the use or safety of any diet, procedure or treatment mentioned in this book. The author or publisher is not responsible for errors or omissions that may exist.

Warning

The Book is for informational purposes only and before taking on any diet, treatment or medical procedure, it is recommended to consult with your primary health care provider.

Our books are available at

1. Amazon.com
2. Barnes and Noble
3. Itunes
4. Kobo
5. Smashwords
6. Google Play Books

Table of Contents

Preface 4

Introduction 5

Chapter 1 - Collecting water 6

Discerning Filtration and Purification 7

Chapter 2 - Filteration Techniques.. 8

Building a water filter... 10

Chapter 3 - Purification techniques... 11

Boiling 11

Filtration or purification pumps 11

Purification drops and tablets 12

Make an evaporation trap in the ground. 12

Turning urine and salt water into drinkable water............... 13

Solar still... 13

Chapter 4 - Choose Your Snow Wisely.................................... 15

How to melt snow the right way.. 16

Does the water from snow need to be purified? 16

Chapter 5 - Different Approaches to Hydration 18

Chapter 6 - Minimising Water Loss... 20

Conclusion 23

Author Bio.. 26

Publisher 37

Preface

Water is a part of life that is as important as your most vital organs. Without water, you cannot perform your day to day activities as none of your internal organs will cooperate with you. Water is the support system on which your body relies.

Now what this book is here to guide you in, is how to find this source of life in survival situations and make sure that it is pure and clean, and ready to be consumed. In our daily city dwellings, we have organized our structure and finding water isn't an issue. The purification has also been simplified by the existence of various filtration equipments in the market. Boiling on stoves is a readily used technique as well, but when you are out in the wilderness none of these homely technologies are your companions there.

The book starts off with giving you helping points on how to cope with the limited availability of water. Then it moves on to helping you to find water in all different scenarios. After all, how can you purify water when you have none of it available to you.

After clearing out the confusion between filtration and purification, we provide you with several techniques for both these steps to consuming safe and healthy water.

Hydration of the body is a must and whether you find water or not, the demands of the body have to be fulfilled. Therefore, we provide you with other sources that can replenish your hydration needs, providing you with different hydration techniques as well.

Lastly, we urge you to focus on the importance of preplanning your expeditions and camping trips. You have to always be prepared for the worst case scenarios and be fully aware of the map you are about to take your journey on.

Introduction

Nothing, I repeat nothing, is more important than water for humans to live on this planet (well excluding oxygen though that's obvious). Your body is made up of around 60-80% water and you cannot hope to continue performing your daily chores with the same efficiency if you don't find enough water. Certainly the amount of usage of water varies depending upon the climate and activities you are involved in, but its presence is always required.

In a moderate climate with low levels of activity, approximately 2 liters of water is required daily for a 160 lb person. Certainly when the climate changes or the level of activity turns to exercise, you need to increase this amount simultaneously. The first sign of dehydration may be discerned through the color of the urine. A normal hydrated body produces a pale yellow color, but a dehydrated body produces urine that is darker in color. To make sure that the body doesn't dehydrate you need to not only meet the required quantity of water, but you also have to make sure that the water is clean.

The reason why you constantly need to drink water is because your body continuously releases liquids and you need to maintain those levels. The release of liquids from your body is in the form of urination, sweating, excretion, and respiration. The liquids are released so that the toxins can be removed from your body and proper hydration makes this happen along with redistributing the nutrients in the body. Water also provides the pathway for electrical impulses to travel through nerve and brain cells to activate the muscles. The brain in itself is made up of 80% water.

Chapter 1 - Collecting water

I know in a survival situation the first concern that you all will be having is probably the availability of water, rather than observing how clean the water is. True, I would also drink from an unclean source if I was at the point of quitting, but clearly the situations may vary. On the other hand, it is always important to learn these tips so that you can perform them to make sure that that drink doesn't prove to be your last in this world.

Now first, here are a few great methods to make your water arrangements and this water is clean and drinkable. All you need is plastic bags, bottles and handkerchiefs.

i.   Wrap a plastic bag tightly around a branch of a tree. Trees are great sources of water and you will get water collected in that plastic bag through the process of condensation. The water won't be too much, but you have something.

ii.   Take a branch full of leaves and place it inside the water bottle. The process remains the same, condensation. This will make sure that at the end of your day, you have 1/3 of a cup to drink.

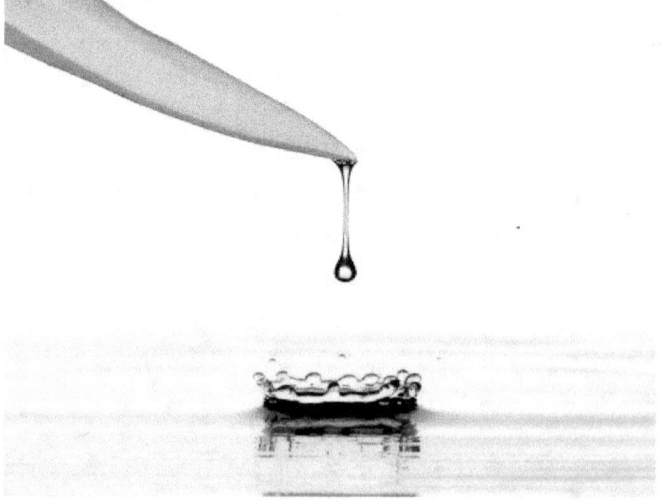

iii.   Rain water is the prime time to catch water. Use sheets to collect the rain water. Roll them up at the end and place water carefully in your bottles.

Discerning Filtration and Purification

There is a difference between water that is filtered and water that is purified. Filtered water mean that the water is free from visible impurities like dirt, insects and plants etc. The purified water is one from which all invisible impurities have been removed as well. So the steps are like this; the water has to be filtered first and then it has to be purified. After these processes the water can be safely enjoyed.

Chapter 2 - Filteration Techniques

After clearing up the confusion between filtration and purifctaon, let us now take each of them, one by one, and learn more about their aid to us.

Okay, so the first step to filtration is called a 35mm film container water filter. The process would require two plastic water bottle water caps and white disposable coffee filters or a piece of white cloth. After making sure that you have all these items, take a sharp blade and make a circular hole at the bottom of the plastic film container. The hole should neither be too big nor too small. Then take one of the plastic bottle caps, and with a pointed knife, make a bunch of small holes in it and place it within the film container. Lastly, place the white cloth inside the film container. You are ready to start filtering.

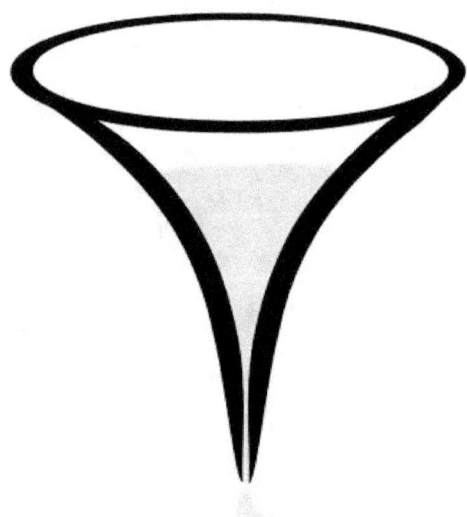

Now it must have entered your mind, why did we need the other bottle cap? Well the other cap has its use. It's basically to squeeze out the last few remaining drops, and more importantly, for covering the hole after you have removed the other cap from the bottle so that you can keep it clean when not using it. When the water starts dripping slowly or drips with still a discolored appearance, it's time to change the white cloth.

Since it is not possible that all your water sources are like a moving stream or creek, sometimes all you find might be a stagnant pond or a swamp. In this case not only filtration is important but it is also essential that you remove the bad odor and taste from the water.

So what do you need to make this happen? Well the answer is an empty plastic bottle and three socks. If you don't have socks, you may use three cut pieces of clothes.

Step 1: Is to cut the bottle in half and roll up each sock tightly. Turn the top half of the bottle upside down and place the first sock inside it.

Step 2: Is to place some of the black burnt charcoal from a fire on top of the first sock. Make sure that no white ashes get into the bottle.

Step 3: Is to place the second sock inside the bottle and to place non salty sand from a non salty river source. Note that it is important that you do not just place any sand and it has to be non salty.

Step 4: Is to place the last sock inside and add grass to it. The purpose of this concoction is NOT to purify the water, this procedure only removes the foul taste and odor of the water.

The most important part of this filter system is the socks; they should be rolled up very tight. When placed inside the plastic water bottle they should fit comfortably and tight inside.

Now, if you find that the water is free from the foul odor, use a clean sock to filter it. Only use this for clean water, and the procedure may be done with any white cloth.

Another rather more fancy and time consuming method to clean the water requires two large buckets, a cotton (not synthetic but cotton only) cloth and patience.

The idea is to keep the two buckets side by side. One will hold the dirty water and the other will accumulate the filtered water. Keep the end of the bucket containing the contaminated water and tip one side of the roughly cut cotton garment in the bucket. As the water will flow through the threads of the cotton garments and flow into the other bucket (as one end of the cloth is placed there) you will find clean water. As we said, this methodology is indeed quite time consuming although more garments can speed it up.

Building a water filter

You can also make a filter from the cone of a birch bark. To make the cone, use a sharp knife to cut at least 14 inches horizontally and then make a second horizontal cut of the same length exactly below it. After this, cut the vertical marks to join the horizontal ones. Try to pry the bark off in one piece. Start rolling the bark inwards like you roll a newspaper. Roll the bottom end more tightly leaving only a tiny space for the filtered water to go through. The cone has to be filled with a layer of sand, charcoal, and grass. The sand helps in trapping the suspended particles in the water. Charcoal acts in a way that removes the chemical impurities, but according to common belief, it cannot stop all the bacteria. Now it's not necessary that filtering it once will get you the desired results and you may have to pass the filtered water through this process again. You can be the judge for the number of times required. General rule of thumb is that the bigger the bark, the more layers have to be added to it.

The birch bark cone should have a fairly small hole at the bottom. The cone has to be tied together to prevent it from opening. You should also place a few stones right at the bottom; this will help in keeping the filtrate fixed in its place.

Chapter 3 - Purification techniques

Now let's come to the part where the water needs to be purified. After all, filtration alone is not what we require, as it will not serve our purpose of obtaining water fit for drinking.

The following are some easy ways for purifying water out in the wilderness:

Boiling

The easiest way by far to purify water is to boil it. Be it campfire or the open sun, you will always have resources to boil water. The speed of boiling may vary though. Bring water in a pot over a high heat source until you have rolling bubbles, then let the water boil for at least five minutes. Then let it cool down before drinking, or you'll have blister on your lips and tongue.

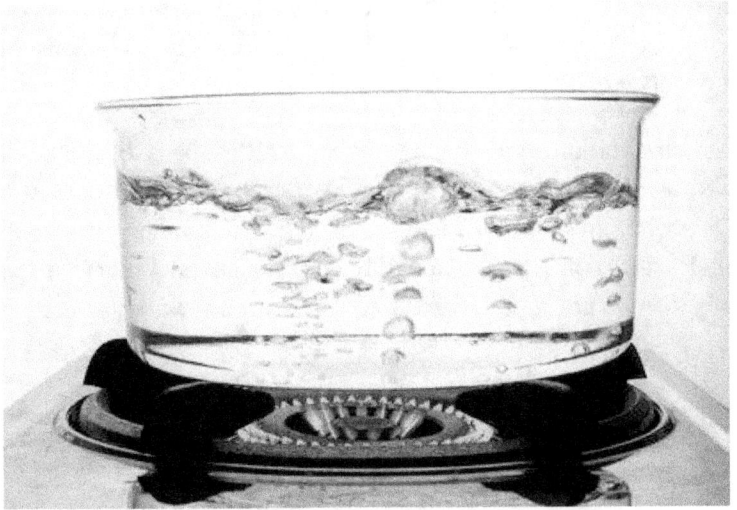

Filtration or purification pumps

If you go to a camping and outdoors supply store, you'll find many different kinds of pumps with filters and purifiers. This purification is done through a process of squeezing water through a ceramic or a charcoal filter and treating it with chemicals.

With recent technology, some hi-tech water bottles have this process built into them. The purification process happens as you squeeze or suck water directly into your mouth.

Purification drops and tablets

A simple method of purifying wild water is by dropping in a couple of purification tablets or drops. The most common chemical used is iodine, but chlorine or potassium permanganate is also effective. Let the chemicals treat the water for at least 20 minutes before consuming, and mix it with powdered mixes to make it taste better, because these tablets do ruin it. These bottles, once opened, have to be utilized within a year because as they come into contact with air, these tablets lose their potency to treat water. Use a pair of tweezers to place them in the water, since the oil from your hands can deteriorate these tablets as well. The Aquamira water treatment drops are ideal for survival trips. This powerful formula of chlorine dioxide kills 99% of all pathogens and purifies 30 gallons of water with just 1 ounce of Aquamira in the liquid form.

This water purification straw can purify up to 120 gallons of drinkable water with one straw. This is a perfect survival water purification method that can fit in your pocket and is easily accessible when out hunting or hiking. The SureAqua Purification Straw is a handy item for anyone's survival pack or emergency kit. Do not drink directly out of a Stream without one.

Make an evaporation trap in the ground.

All of the previous methods require you to carry water or have a water source nearby. Now what would you do if that is not the case? According to researchers you can pull moisture out of the earth by digging a hole in the ground and inserting a container on the bottom. Cover the hole with plastic so that no moisture escapes, and put a small rock in the center of the cover so that there's a dip in the center. When the water evaporates from the ground upwards, it condenses on the cover and drips down into the container. This is certainly not the fastest way, but hey, better something than going thirsty.

Turning urine and salt water into drinkable water.

Yes, there is a way from which you can turn these unhealthy sources of water into ones that can be consumed. What you require is two containers with lids and a metal rod to connect them. The container with the impure water should be placed on fire and the other container should be placed on a rock or a slightly higher ground. The metal rod should now connect these two containers. What happens is that the pure vapors of water will travel through the rod and fall safely into the empty container. This water can be safely consumed.

Solar still

A solar still or a distillatory is equipment used to purify liquids. What basically happens is that a heat source is used to create vapors. The vapors condense as they cool down and turn that liquid into its pure form. This is what we will teach you to perform to safely consume water in the wilderness.

Solar stills are being used in countries where pure water is not in abundance. There are different types of survival solar stills or vapor stills. Usually the pit solar still is used in survival.

The first step is that you have to carefully analyze your surroundings. If the ground is very dry, a solar still will produce less water, but if you can find a dried creek or added vegetation, the quantity of water generated can increase.

A sheet of plastic can be your savior, and it is not only required for this solar still procedure, you can also use it for shelter and as protection for your food. We shall make use of the heat from the sun and the moisture of the soil. Increased vegetation like a crushed cactus or adding unclean water into the pit would also help.

The shape of the pit can either be square or like the letter "V". Note that you may use a pit box that does not have vegetation, only the amount of water generated would be low. Simply place a small bowl in the center of the pit and cover it with clear plastic. Sand can be used as an anchor for the plastic, or you may also use stones. Stones can be placed right above the bowl in the precise middle of it. Now, as the water evaporates and condenses, this cycle will generate water for you. The common tips include a larger pit with preferably vegetations with added unclean water like urine etc. to speed up evaporation.

Chapter 4 - Choose Your Snow Wisely

Snow is a safe source to drink water from; of course you might have other survival worries, but not water. You want to choose the cleanest snow possible for your water needs. A good start is to avoid collecting snow that has any color. Fresh fallen snow is the safest, of course. The longer snow sits on the ground the more horrible stuff that falls on it and is absorbed from the layers of snow beneath.

Choose snow far from game trails, water sources, and from any waste material. Find clean snow away from trees to avoid snow with bird droppings and other materials falling from trees. Dig beneath the surface of the new snow to find the cleaner snow.

Avoid all "colored" snow:

Did you have you any idea that snow sometimes comes in colors? You're no doubt familiar with yellow snow, but how about red, green, or brown? If the snow isn't nice and white and fresh, please avoid it.

- "Yellow" snow requires no explanation, right?

- "Red" or "Watermelon" snow always contains algae that thrives in freezing water.

- "Green" and "Brown" snow produced by algae are also seen.

When you find the perfect snow, gather it in a small tarp or stuff sack and haul it back to camp. This conserves your energy by making one trip to the "good" snow field.

If you boil the water, more will evaporate through steam, of course. The yield is approximately 43% of the packed snow volume. Your mileage may vary.

Ice is denser than snow and would produce more water through melting. However, ice may contain harmful bacteria that could be released upon melting. So, unless you plan to boil the water produced from ice, just use fresh snow instead.

How to melt snow the right way

The snow-melting process seems like a no-brainer, but there is a right way to do it.

Contrary to what you might think, if you don't pay attention while melting the snow, you can burn water, too. What actually happens is that the water in the pot evaporates and leaves the snow just sitting there, thus scorching the bottom of the pot. The pot smells horrible and the water tastes like burning tires.

The Process:

- Incorrect: Pack snow into a pot and put it on the fire. Avoid it.

- Correct: Put about an inch of water in the cook pot and heat it. Start adding a little snow and stir as it melts. This takes time.

If when you add the snow to the pot it absorbs all of the heated water, then you didn't start with enough water in the pot. Add more water now or you will end up scorching the water because of the lack of liquid present. You'll also want to use a lid on the pot to conserve heat, but open the lid to stir the water as the snow melts.

Does the water from snow need to be purified?

Not necessarily. If you've chosen a snow source wisely, purification isn't as critical. Melting the snow without boiling should be all that is needed. Even fresh snow has stuff in it that was picked up in the sky when it was forming. It's the same stuff that ends up in bodies of water when it rains. Stuff like dust particles, pollen grains, seeds and plants are carried by winds and deposited with snow on the surface.

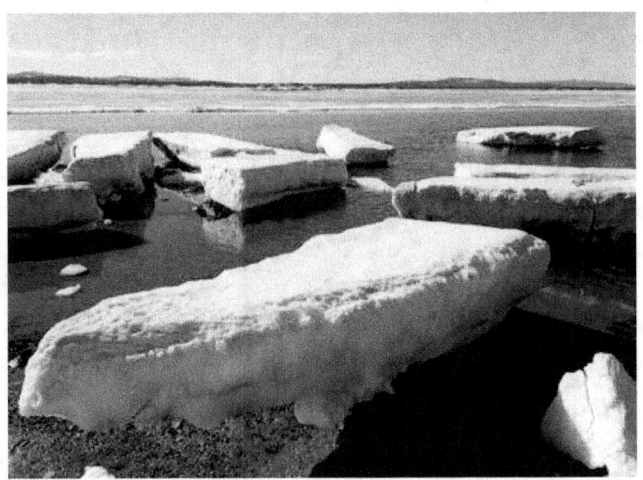

Snow and ice (so long as it's not sea ice!) can provide a good, readily available source of clean water in the winter. One thing that is of utmost importance is that you should never eat snow or ice. Doing so will lower your body temperature while not doing as much for hydration as melted snow will.

Chapter 5 - Different Approaches to Hydration

Pre-Hike Hydration:

Most of us are slightly dehydrated most of the time, even when you don't feel the need for a glass of water. Therefore, drink extra water at home a day or two before the hike and on the way to the trailhead. At least start your hike fully hydrated and that will be a big plus. Experts believe that maximum in-the-field hydration will occur this way.

Trailhead Hydration:

Drink lots of water from known clean sources at the trailhead, it may come from a clean spring or your reserves. Do the same upon returning. It is a good way to moderate the almost universal dehydration effect from longer, more vigorous hikes. Remember, it is always better to drink before you get thirsty. This practice should result both in getting ahead of hydration needs and carrying less water.

Calculate Water Needs:

Treat and carry only as much water as you actually need to get to the next dependable water source. These amounts are based on factors like previous experience and knowledge of the area. It is very difficult to calculate actual water needs. This often results in either carrying excess weight or getting really thirsty when one miscalculates.

Carry Extra Water:

As a matter of habit, treat as much water as you can comfortably carry. One can never predict exact water needs. Be conservative and prepare for any emergencies. This is always helpful when you are the group leader and have to analyze the weakness and hydration levels of your team.

Cameling:

Tank up from the highest quality natural sources while on the trail; this is what is referred to as cameling. One exception is that if one is perspiring a lot it is better to drink smaller amounts often and to refill electrolytes to avoid any medical issues.

Eating Stops Based on Water Availability:

Do not necessarily camp where there is water. This will not be the correct approach. Keep moving forward. Leave camp and hike to a water source and stop for breakfast. Then hike to water sources for lunch stops. Similarly for dinner and after that hike some more to a camping spot carrying only enough water to rehydrate a bit during the night hours.

Keep in mind that this approach works only if water sources are relatively frequent and hydration needs are moderate. If hydration needs are greater, then carrying plenty of water becomes a necessity.

Chapter 6 - Minimising Water Loss

Water can be found at the base of the cliff and mountains, trapped between the rocks. Or if you are in a desert, every green thing means the presence of water and similarly in low lying vegetation areas its presence may be noted. In any survival situation where water is short in supply, the first step is to protect and conserve water already in the body. This is what we want you to focus on initially before taking you on the journey to learn ways to purify the water that you find.

1. Cover any areas of exposed skin as soon as you can. This protects against sunburn, which would otherwise lead to more water loss from damaged cells. In hot conditions, it also helps in reducing evaporation of sweat from the body, which helps in reducing the need to replace bodily fluids lost from sweating. Loose clothing is better than tighter fitting clothes in this situation because it traps the relatively still air around the body, thereby insulating it from the external temperature. The air that is trapped, gains humidity from evaporated perspiration and then slows the evaporation rate.

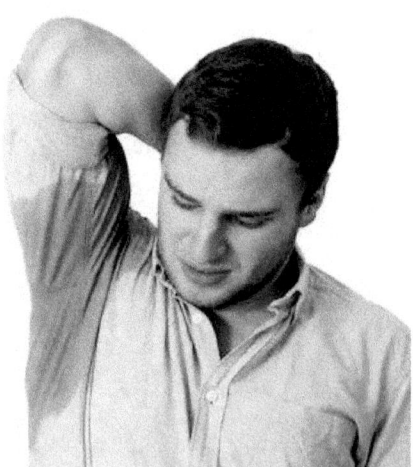

2. Regardless of the climate, try to breathe through the nose and cover the face with a towel, shirt ,or other cloth to reduce water loss through breathing. Grass can be chewed on to reduce thirst. Keep the mouth closed and talk only when necessary.

3. Try to stay in the shade during the day and minimize movement to reduce dehydration caused by direct sunlight. Sit or lay a little bit above the ground surface using anything that is available, including fallen trees, rocks, leaves or anything else that's available. Even if it's just a few inches it will help provide a layer of insulation and slow dehydration.

4. In hotter conditions, avoid traveling or other types of strenuous work during the hottest parts of the day. If you have to move, do it as slowly as possible to keep body heat generation to a minimum. This will help to reduce the body's indulgence of fluid as it tries to maintain a low body temperature.

5. In warmer conditions, drink during the cool hours of the early mornings, late afternoon, or evening. Your body uses calories to warm any water that's ingested. In cooler conditions try to let your water warm in the sun or near the fire, because drinking cold water in an already cold environment can cause chills.

6. Don't swallow large amounts of water. It is better to drink before you get thirsty and feel dehydrated. When you feel your mouth getting dry you are already about 4% dehydrated. Also, the body can only process little amounts of water at a time, so giving breaks between drinking is making the most efficient usage of water.

7. Sea water or other waste water can be used to wet your clothes and cool you down and help to reduce sweating. If you build a survival still you can use this water to make clean drinking water as well. DO NOT DRINK SALTWATER, this will bring DEATH more quickly than drinking nothing at all.

8. When you have scarce water resources you should also eat less, because the water inside you will be used up more quickly for the process of digestion.

9. You have to be careful of Urban Water Survival Myths. Often when you are desperate, you will have a greater tendency to make bad decisions which can land you in more poor conditions. Remember your basics and the above principles and you will be better off than trying dangerous schemes to try and rehydrate yourself.

10. You may have to measure what little water is available, but if you can limit fluid loss, you can make the water you have last longer. This extra time and conservation of resources will allow further opportunity to find or create another water source.

Conclusion

Clear flowing water coming from somewhere without people, manmade things, or apparent signs of pollution are best. If you come across a spring while outdoors, take advantage of it and top off your water bottles.

Lakes, ponds, and rivers are less ideal. The first two are stagnant, which may mean increased levels of bacteria, while large rivers are typically full of pollution. Be especially wary after any flooding or if the river flows from or through a population center, under a road or around any construction, on its way to you.

If you can't find a water source, start walking downhill. Not only is that an excellent strategy for finding your way back, but topping this advantage you can even find water. Look for dark patches in the landscape, especially on rocky hills and any group of vegetation that stands out in a low area.

Honestly though, don't put yourself in the kind of situation where you need to find water. Plan trips in areas where it's available or, if you're traveling through the desert on a dirt bike, map out where it's available ahead of time. A little bit of planning and you'll never find yourself hoping you had never taken this journey.

Now, since in survival situations it is not always essential that you may find water, you have to find other ways to keep yourself hydrated. You cannot solely rely on finding water again.

The most basic thing is to use the moisture in plants, fruits animals and fish to keep you hydrated.

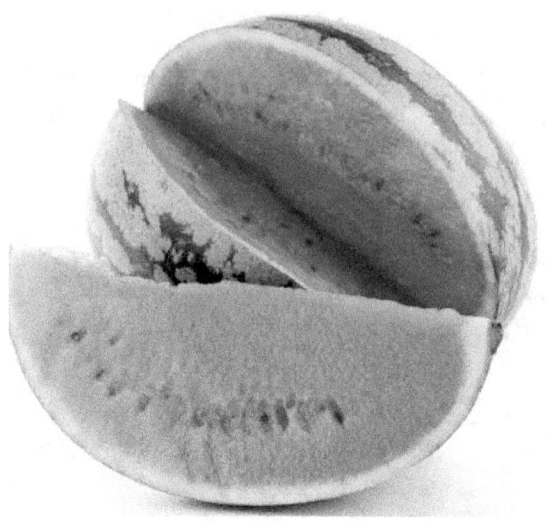

Edible berries, palm fruits, and prickly pears are great sources for moisture. Remember to spit out the pits afterwards. Other Fruits provide an excellent source for water. Watermelon is 90% water, so it ranks highest on the list. Oranges, grapefruit, and melons like cantaloupe and honeydew are also strong contenders. Vegetables, though not as full of water as fruit, can also provide a nutrient-rich water source. Stick with celery, cucumbers, tomatoes, green peppers, and Romaine lettuce. Green coconuts provide you with water and the brown ones with milk. But one thing has to be kept in mind, and that is excess of these water sources may cause diarrhea. Tap into a fig tree. Just make sure you have a tube and container absolutely prepared because the water issue is about to be resolved.

There are plenty of hidden sources of water in your diet. If you want to tap into these foods, reach for oatmeal and yogurt. Make sure you pack them in good quantities for your journey.

Pull open plant stalks, thick vines, and bamboos, as they have loads of plant moisture in them as well. Although you should keep in mind that their roots are generally toxic, so you should not drink directly from them. Some of the cacti plants contain water stored in them. Make sure that initially you cut off the spines before making an attempt to access the moisture of the plant.

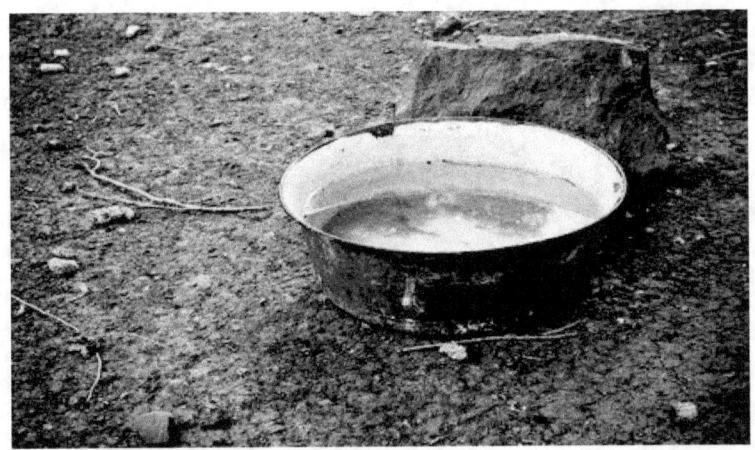

A rainstorm is natures way of being kind to you. Lay out large leaves, sea shells, and bamboo pieces cut in halves. Capture as much water as you can and store it. You may also dig a hole and line it with plastic.

Remember all these tips so if you are ever in a survival situation, you can make it until help arrives.

Author Bio

Muhammad Usman is a distinguished medical graduate of Allama Iqbal medical college (AIMC). He is a professional writer who has been in the field for more than 4 years. During this time he has produced 10,000+ articles, blogs, and eBooks on various niches related to diseases, health, fitness, nutrition and well-being. He is a regular contributor to several journals related to medicine and surgery. He is the editor of several journals and newspapers.

Check out some of the other JD-Biz Publishing books

Gardening Series on Amazon

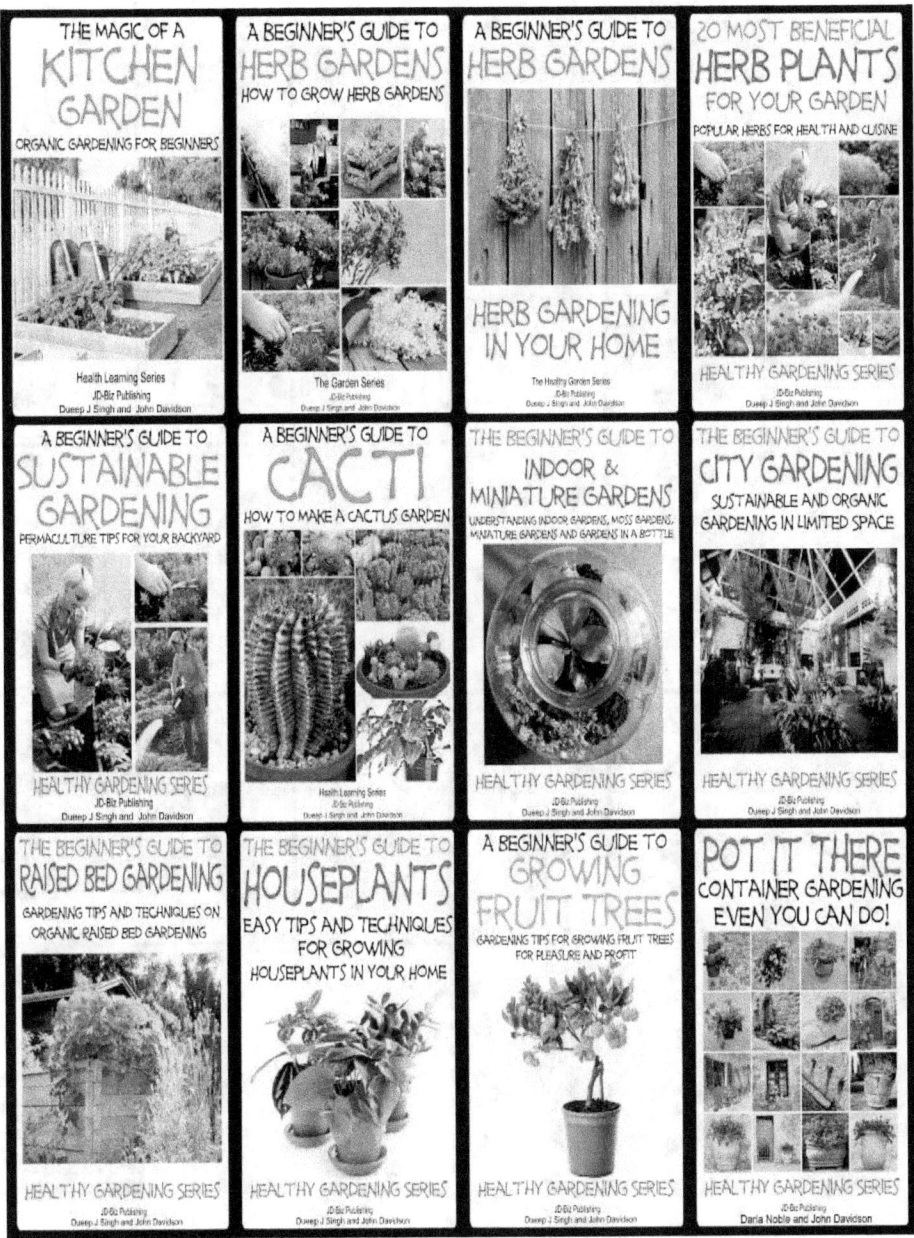

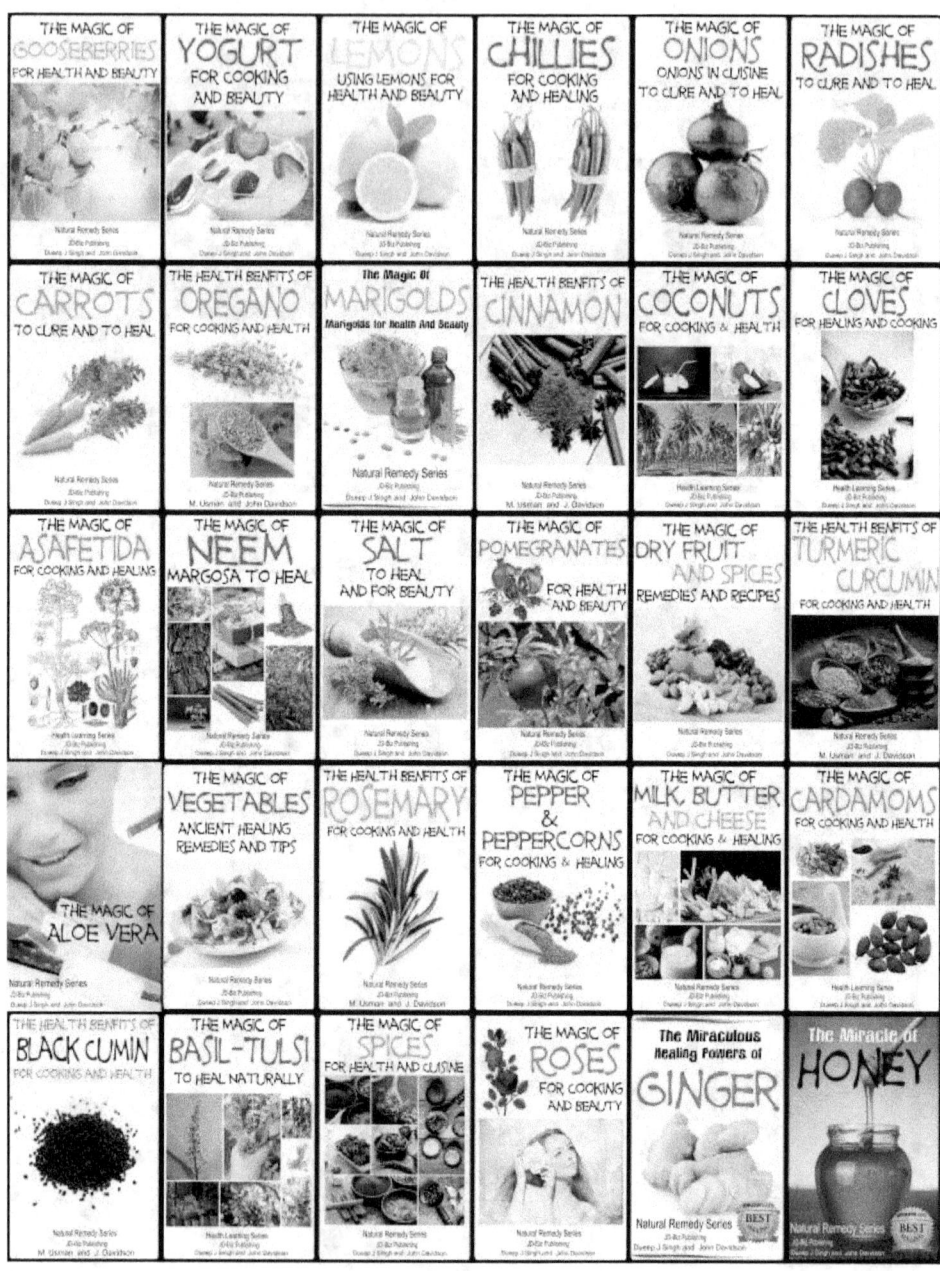

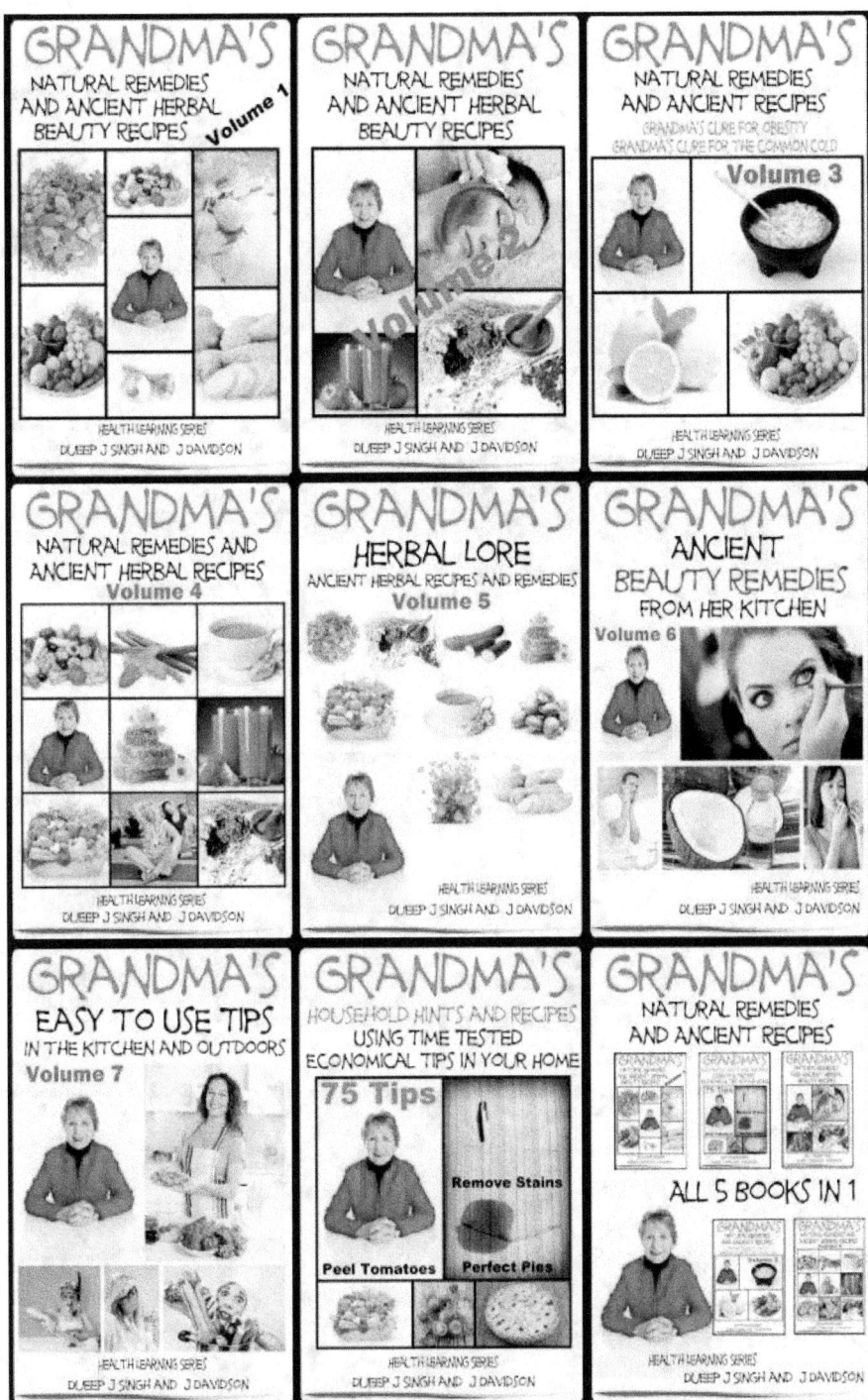

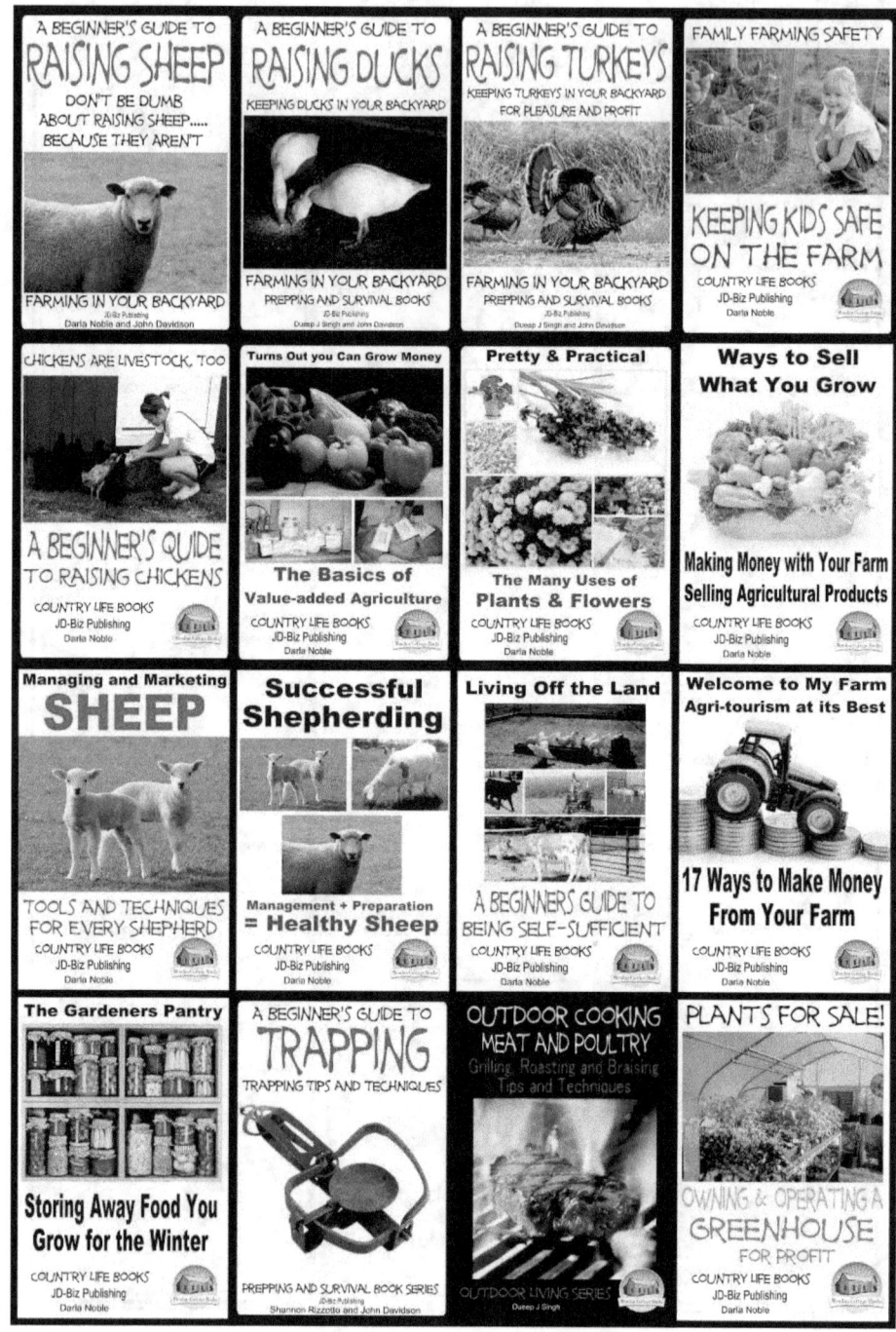

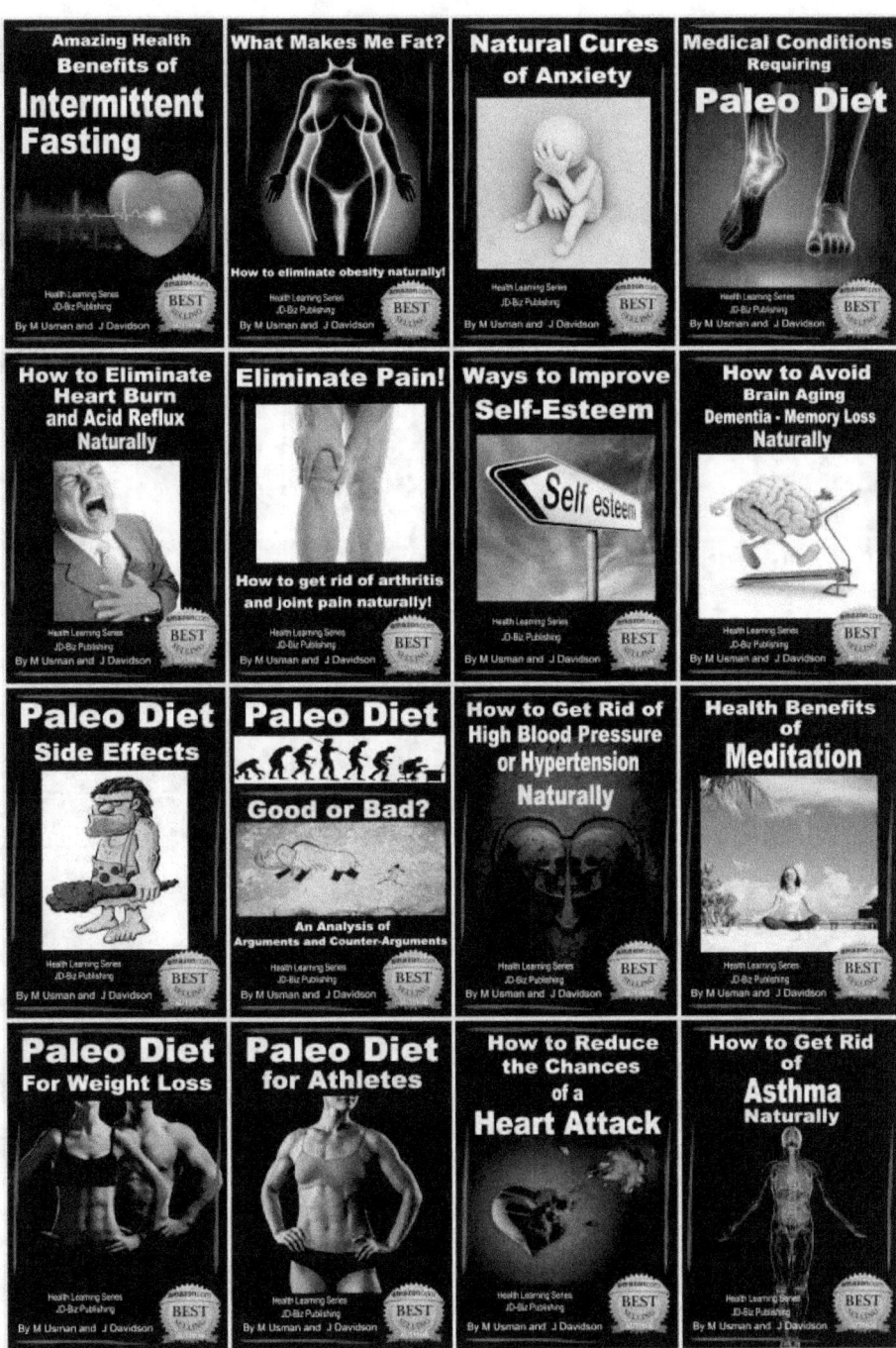

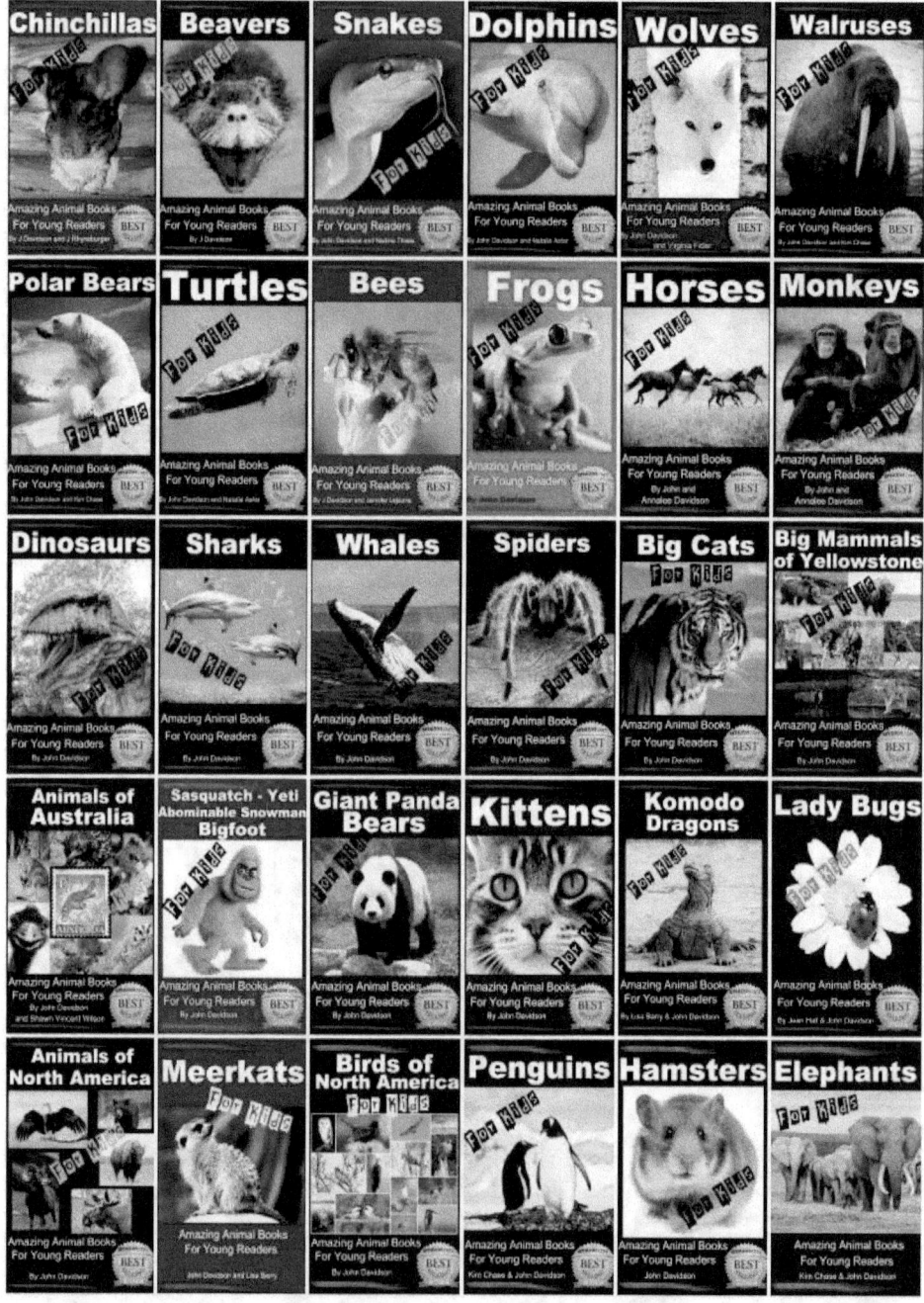

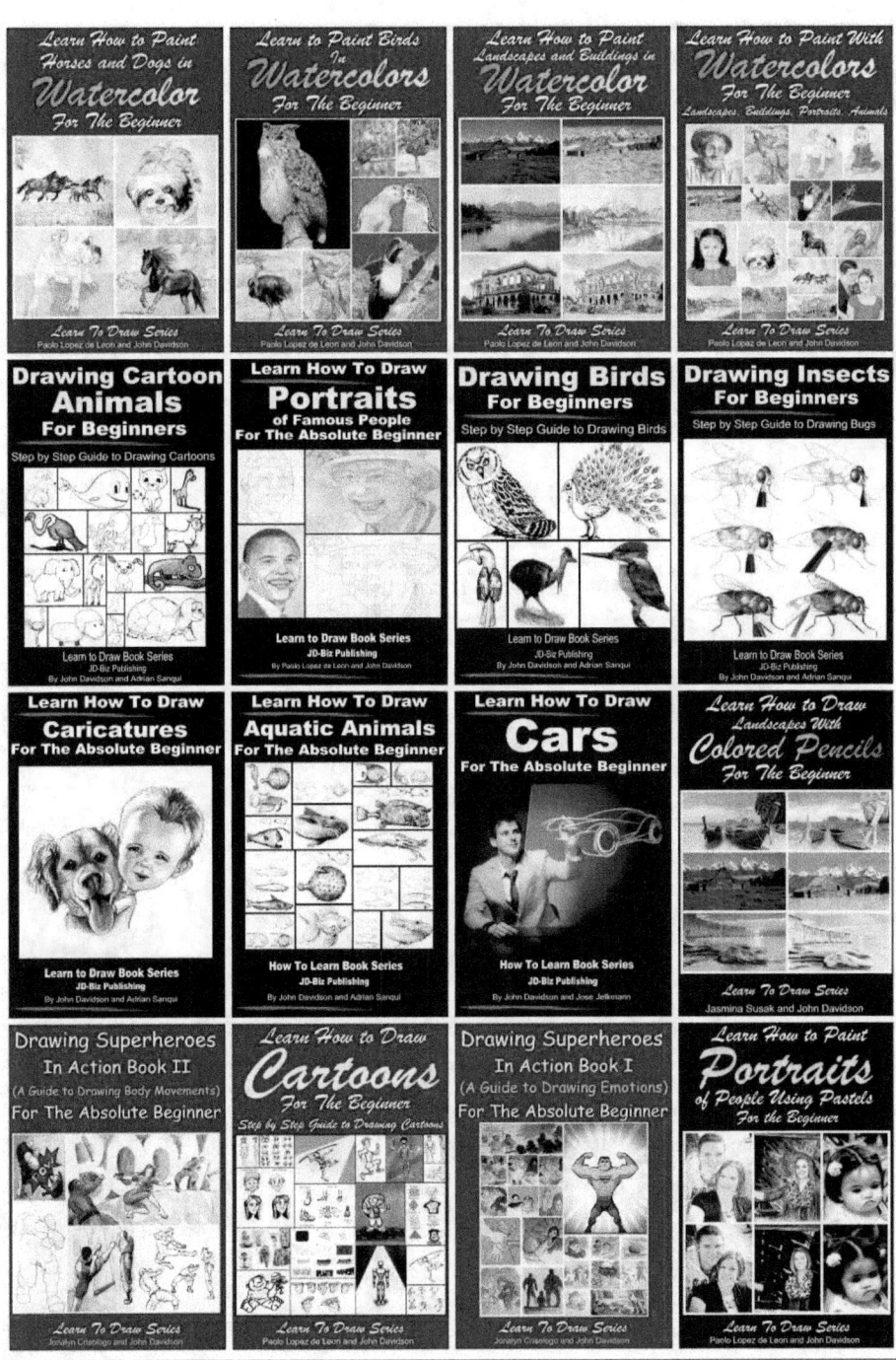

How to Build and Plan Books

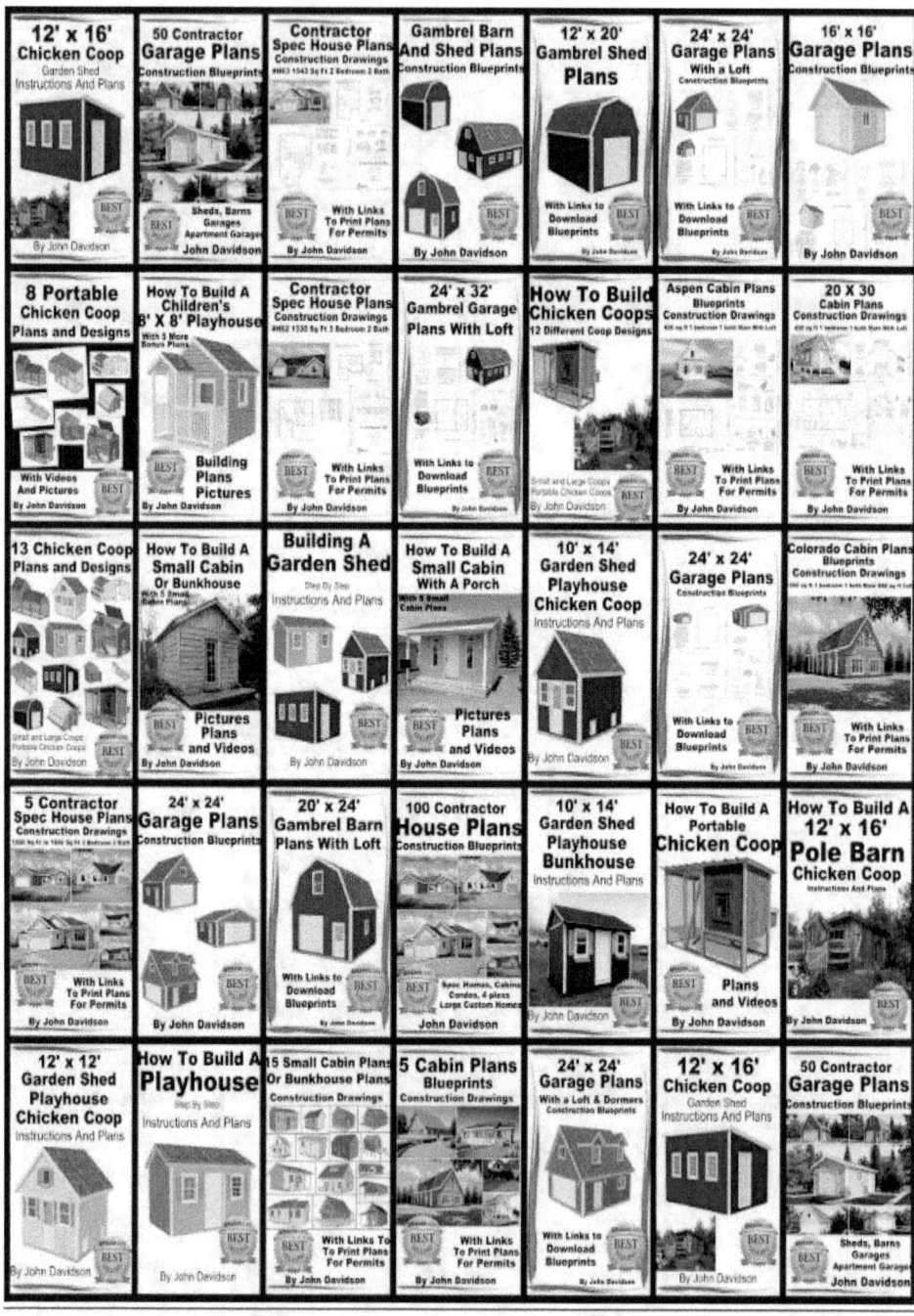

Entrepreneur Book Series

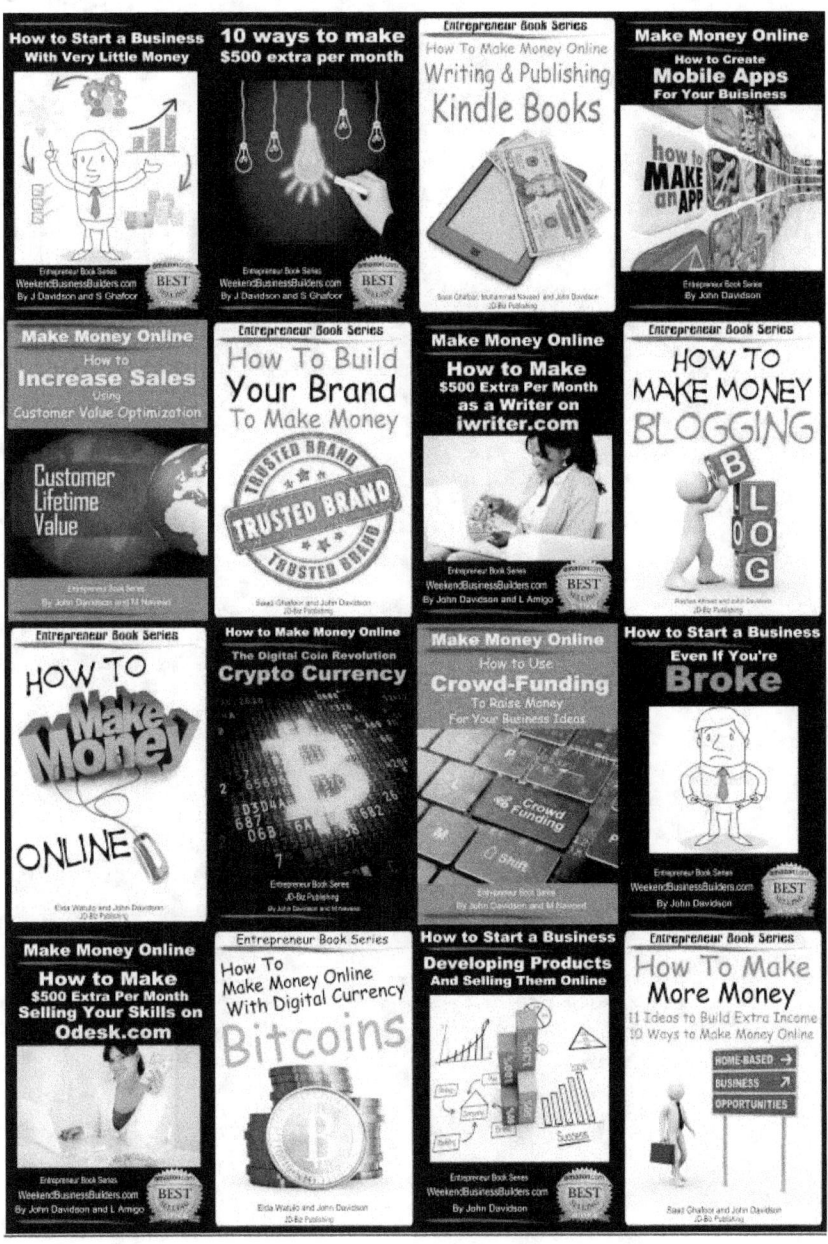

Our books are available at

1. Amazon.com

2. Barnes and Noble

3. Itunes

4. Kobo

5. Smashwords

6. Google Play Books

Publisher

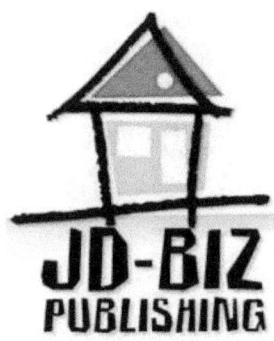

JD-Biz Corp

P O Box 374

Mendon, Utah 84325

http://www.jd-biz.com/

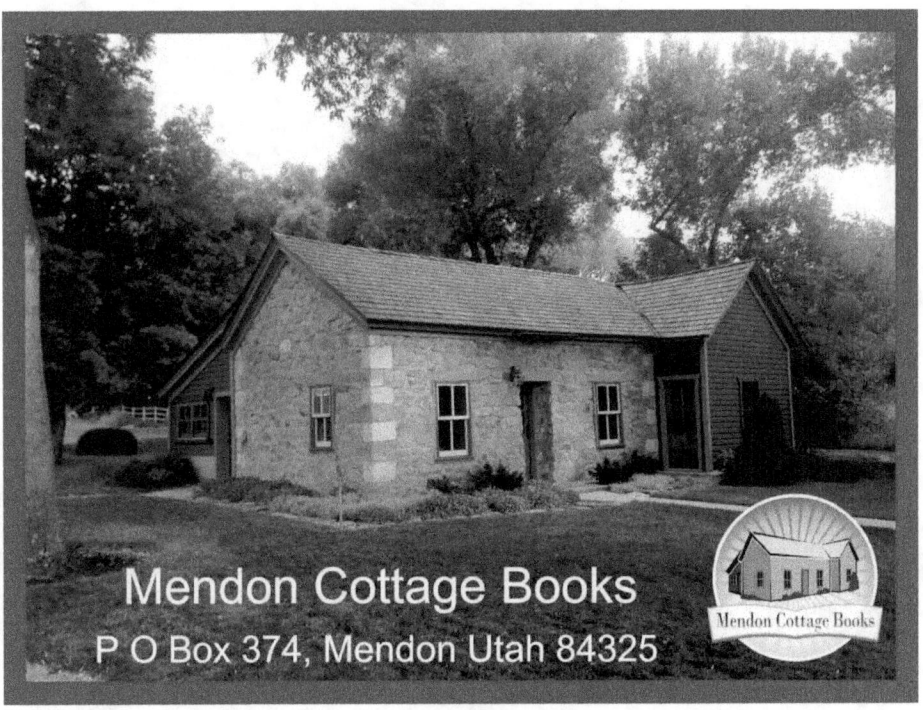

www.ingramcontent.com/pod-product-compliance
Lightning Source LLC
Chambersburg PA
CBHW061937280526
45787CB00004B/1634